I0419818

The Lean And Clean Diet

Dieting secrets and over 30 recipes to get lean and stay healthy

Liam Abby

Introduction

Hey,

Thank you for buying this book, I know you are going to love it!

I wrote the book to prove that losing weight is not as complicated as the fitness industry is trying to make you believe, with all these supplements and fat burners…

Losing weight is in part a matter of training, and partly a nutritional balance, this involves choosing foods high in water and fiber and contains little fat especially bad. You can do all the crunches and the cardio workouts you want, your abs will be always hidden under fat if the pizza and hamburgers are the mainstay of your diet. If you want to lose weight, there is no magic solution you have to follow a simple and proper nutrition; we have prepared a comprehensive scheme of fat loss diet and lot of easy and delicious recipes to help you reach your goals.

The Fat Loss Plan

Everybody who wants to lose weight must have a plan to attack, it can't be done just like that, randomly. In this chapter i'll show you where to start and how to plan your fat loss diet.

Setting a goal

The first step in any fat loss diet is to evaluate the weight you need to lose; it's motivating to regularly track progress. What matters is to be realistic and not try to lose too much too soon. Experts say that it is better not to lose more than 2-3lbs a week because a brutal drop in calories leads to lot of muscle loss.

For a man, a fat level between 8 and 15% is considered satisfactory. Most people who are near the low values of these ranges are top athletes in competition form and is rarely desirable or reasonable to stay this dry year around. Because of the difficulties encountered for accurate fat rate, the simplest is to use a tape measure and measure waist circumference. In general, the loss of 1 inch around the waist is equivalent to an overall loss of 4 pounds of fat: it is a good rule of thumb that applies to both men and women to calculate its fat.

Lose 20 pounds of fat is losing 5 inches waistline rather than 20 pounds would indicate as your scales

The importance of muscles to lose weight

On any fat loss plan it is important to keep and as much muscles as possible. Muscle tissue is an active tissue that needs and uses calories just to continue being. Some studies have shown that 1 pound of muscle can burn up to 50 calories per day by simply existing. This means that if you gain 10 lbs of muscle you can eat 500 more calories per day and still lose fat. This is just one of many reasons why it is so important to preserve muscle mass when burning fat. . So, if you lose 5 inches on your waist and 30 pounds (which is the norm for most people who lose weight without exercise) you will also have lost about 10 pounds of "Muscles". Some loss of muscle mass is usually difficult to avoid, but it can be reduced significantly by losing weight more gradually, consuming at least 1.0 gram of protein per pound of body weight.

Record what you eat

Each individual is different and the number of calories a person can burn daily can vary widely depending on the level of activity. That is why it is better to write down everything you eat for ten consecutive days minimum, plus snacks and the total amount of each food. This somewhat tedious exercise is still the safest way to determine caloric intake to observe to maintain or decrease their body weight. Note the retail food taken for at least ten days allows awareness and this method really puts you face the reality of what you eat and especially quantities.

In fact, keep a nutrition diary or diet often helps improve eating habits. Enter "candy" and other types of sweets encourage your thinking: it's an eye opening experience! Once you know the number of calories you tend to eat each day, reduce this total by about 30% to make the first step in your slimming special diet. It will be about 300-500 fewer calories per day for someone who weighs over 180 pounds, with a low risk of losing muscles.

Macronutrients

Calories: Calories are units of measure assigned to foods to show how much energy it contains. Your body consume a certain number of calories as energy every day.

If you consume more calories than you burn, the excess will be stored as body fat. If you consume less than you expend everyday your body will have to use stored fat to meet energy needs, it's that simple.

This is the accurate formula to calculate how much calories you need to burn   fat:

Body weight x 16 = Daily caloric intake

Protein: Proteins are very important molecules to the human body. On any fat loss plan protein is absolutely essential to maintaining muscle mass. The body prefers to use protein for building muscle tissue rather than to use it for energy. Glycogenesis result in protein breakdown to use it for energy and this is not preferred when trying to maintain muscle mass .Not only does this process result in the breakdown of muscle tissue but protein also yields less energy per unit than carbohydrates or fat. So protein is best used as a building block of muscles, rather than being used for energy.

To calculate you daily protein needs you can use this formula:

Body weight x 1.0 gram = Daily protein intake

Fats: Fats are essential molecules that cannot be ignored in a fat loss plan because of the important roles they play in many different bodily processes. Fat is the most energy dense nutrient whereas protein and carbs both contain 4 calories per gram, fat contains 9 calories per gram. An important function of fat is its role in the production of testosteron which is an anabolic hormone that accelerate fat burning .Fat acids are a substrate for cholesterol, meaning that fatty acids must be available to create cholesterol. This is important because cholesterol is eventually converted to testosterone. If fat intake is too low testosterone production will drop to low levels which results in loss of muscle mass and fat gain.

The important thing is to decrease fat intake when trying to lose weight, but at the same time make sure daily intake does not drop so low that testosterone levels will be affected.

To calculate fat intake:

Body weight x 0.5 = Daily fat intake

Carbohydrates: Carbohydrates are broken down into glucose which is the primary energy source that fuels the body. Glucose is converted into glycogen and stored within muscle tissue where it is held until it is ready to be used during effort.

In the absence of sufficient carbs, your body will have to convert amino acids to glucose for energy. These amino acids may normally be stored as proteins, so you could say that carbs are anti-catabolic because they are protein sparing. Carbohydrates are essential to keeping a fast metabolism leptin and other fat burning hormones are directly related to carbohydrate intake and body fat levels, leptin is a fat burning hormone that serves many functions. One of the most important functions is the control of energy expenditure. When food intake, and most notably carb intake is high, leptin levels will be high. This sends signals to you body that it is in a fed state and this can cause your metabolism to remain high.

When carbs are low, leptin levels will lower. This will send signals to the body that energy intake is low and the metabolism must be lowered to compensate for the lack of incoming energy. When carbs are kept in the diet it will help keep levels of leptin and other fat burning hormones even when total calorie intake is low. When muscle cells are depleted this tells your body that food is in short supply and it will take action by lowering fat burning hormones as you see, carbohydrates must remain in the diet for optimal fat loss.

Carbohydrate calculating:

Body weight x 1.5 = Daily carbohydrates intake

Drink a lot of water

For years, dieters have been drinking lots of water as a weight loss strategy. While water doesn't have any magical effect on weight loss, substituting it for higher calorie beverages can certainly help.

"What works with weight loss is if you choose water or a non-caloric beverage over a caloric beverage and/or eat a diet higher in water-rich foods that are healthier, more filling, and help you trim calorie intake," says Penn State researcher Barbara Rolls, PhD.

Don't forget fruits and vegetables

They are rich in vitamins, minerals, fibers and because of their favorable effect on health has been demonstrated. They have a protective role in preventing diseases appear in adulthood, such as cancers, cardiovascular disease, obesity, diabetes ... Most importantly they offer an incredible variety of flavors, everything that it takes to combine health and enjoyment.

So try to eat 5 servings of fruit and / or vegetables, Ex: 3 servings of fruit and two vegetables 4 vegetables and fruit ... and if you can eat more, it's even better! The ideal is to alternate between fruit and vegetable varieties to diversify and integrate as much as possible in your recipes.

Before we get to cooking

Before we get to delicious recipes we will talk about common mistakes people do when trying to lose weight and I'll give you the most effective tips, and secrets about fat loss.

Fat loss diet common mistakes

- Brutal reduction in calories:

   You want a fit physique whatever the cost . You are ready to sacrifice everything . So you decide to halve your calorie intake , hoping to transform your physique a few days. It is a serious mistake, because this method is not only bad for health but the body is unlikely to react in the expected way . A high calorie reduction can work against you by slowing your metabolism , engine burning fat . So it is best to create a small deficit and reduce daily calorie intake slowly.

- Total elimination of fats :

   Complete elimination of lipids From a nutritional standpoint , it is dangerous to completely eliminate a type of food : carbohydrate diets zero , zero and zero cholesterol lipid be avoided at all costs. We can control calories by eliminating the bad fats, such as butter, meat tendon , skin and fried chicken. Yet there are many who go too far and eliminates almost all fat foods to try to sculpt their bodies by limiting itself to the lipid-free protein sources such as white fish, egg whites and protein powders and there it is the problem in all this: diets without fat and therefore cholesterol compromise testosterone levels, which can disrupt the body's ability to maintain muscle mass.

- Eliminating carbohydrates :

    There is no doubt that low carbohydrates diets help reduce body fat, but it is not advisable to completely remove carbohydrates. It is better to pay attention to the type of carbohydrates you eat and when their consumption. One of the best methods is to eliminate sugar all meals except breakfast. At breakfast, they are important because they terminate the catabolism caused by fasting during sleep so stopping muscle destruction .

- Too desperate and short sighted :

  Yes I can understand how badly you want to fit into those size 32 waist jeans or that designer dress in a few weeks. However, in the real world you need to be more patient and think of the long term. I am sure you did not pack on 30 pounds in 3 weeks, so why expect to lose it in 3 weeks?

- Trying to be a perfect dieter :

  The big mistake *perfect dieters* make is that they try to follow their programs so strictly that they don't allow themselves any room for mistakes , So to avoid making this big mistake, please forget about being perfect. Don't quit just because you had something you shouldn't have had. Don't push the panic button. Learn from your mistake, move on and stick with it. A good abs diet should always allow cheat days, so you can eat some of your favourite foods or desserts as a *thank you* to yourself for sticking to the program.

Fat loss secrets and tips:

- Spread your meals :

  Gone are the traditional three meals daily whatever the number of calories consumed each day, it is imperative to split equally between 5-6 small meals. Whenever you eat, metabolism increases under the effect of digestion and thermogenesis. Furthermore, by making smaller meals, you are sure not to overeat, otherwise the excess calories are likely to be stored as fat.

- Think protein :

  For the metabolism remains active, it is important to lose fat and not muscle! Since muscle hypertrophy occurs due to amino acids supplied by the proteins, it is imperative to eat every day. Moreover, as the proteins are degraded slowly in the intestine, they are effective against the tautness of the stomach.

  However, we will stick to lean protein sources such as chicken breast and turkey without the skin , tuna, salmon and lean steak . Warning: no abuse because excess protein can also promote fat gain .

- Fibers against fat :

If body fat is your enemy , fibers are the ally : 100% calorie-free, the fibers absorb water through volume effect , they create a feeling of " stomach fullness " that helps curb appetite . The fibers also regulate the insulin levels in the blood , thus contributing an important factor in controlling weight. The best sources of fiber are grains to sound, legumes and oatmeal. Try to consume 25-35 grams of fiber per day.

- Full balanced breakfast :

Eat sufficient protein (30-40 grams), a complex carbohydrate like oatmeal, and a piece of fruit to start your day good and stop the catabolism.

- Be careful of hidden calories :

If you enjoy a glass of juice with your meals or use it to mix your protein shake, watch out for the extra calories. While New York's Pulido suggests the occasional glass may be fine, he reminds you that liquid calories aren't as filling as whole foods, which provide more volume. According to research in the "American Journal of Clinical Nutrition," 37 percent of Americans' total daily calories come from sugar-sweetened drinks, including sodas and fruit juices, yet these calories do little to make you feel full. If you crave something sweet, a whole fruit provides more vitamins, minerals, and fibers, plus you're less likely to eat additional foods because the volume is greater in your digestive system.

- Limit sugar and junk foods :
  Remove all junk foods from your home you may be tempted to overeat, like snack foods and candy. Anything is OK in moderation, and a cheat here and there is fine. Satisfy your sweet tooth occasionally and try to limit your intake of sugar, because excess sugar will be stored as fat.

- Drink green tea :

The interaction between the caffeine in green tea and the catecheins (more specifically EGCG) in green tea, revs up the body's use of calories as energy. Moreover, the combination of caffeine and EGCG found in green tea was further shown in the British journal of nutrition to significantly increase the resting metabolic rate.

The Recipes

Breakfast Recipes

BROCCOLI & FETA OMELET WITH TOAST

This easy breakfast recipe full of fibers, takes just 15 minutes start to finish, packs a one-two punch that will leave you feeling satisfied yet energized.

Ingredients:

- 1 cup chopped broccoli
- 2 large eggs, beaten
- 2 tablespoons feta cheese, crumbled
- 1/4 teaspoon dried dill
- 2 slices rye bread, toasted

Preparation:

Heat a non-stick skillet over medium heat. Coat pan with cooking spray. Add broccoli, and cook 3 minutes then Combine egg, feta, and dill in a small bowl. Add egg mixture to pan ; Cook 3 to 4 minutes; flip omelet and cook 2 minutes or until cooked through. Serve with toast.

SPICED GREEN TEA SMOOTHIE

Green tea is one of the top fat burning foods, thanks to a metabolism-boosting compound known as EGCG. In one study, drinking four cups of green tea a day helped people cut more than six pounds in eight weeks!

Ingredients:

- 3/4 cup strong green tea, chilled
- 1/8 teaspoon cayenne pepper

- Juice of 1 lemon (2-3 TBSP)
- 2 teaspoons agave nectar
- 1 small pear, skin on, cut into pieces
- 2 tablespoons fat-free plain yogurt
- 6-8 ice cubes

BARLEY WITH BANANA & SUNFLOWER SEEDS

Looking for a healthy start to your day? Tired of oatmeal? Switch things up with this crunchy breakfast bowl. The combination of barley and banana provides nearly 8 grams of resistant starch, plus metabolism-boosting fiber, making this an ultra-satisfying morning meal.

Ingredients:

- 2/3 cup water
- 1/3 cup uncooked quick-cooking pearl barley
- 1 banana, sliced
- 1 tablespoon unsalted salted sunflower seeds
- 1 teaspoon honey

Preparation:

Combine 2/3 cup water and barley in a small microwave-safe bowl. Microwave on HIGH 6 minutes , Stir and let stand 2 minutes. Top with banana slices, sunflower seeds, and honey.

BANANA & ALMOND BUTTER TOAST

One slice contains just 280 calories, but it's guaranteed to keep you full until lunchtime.

Ingredients:

- 1 tablespoon almond butter
- 1 slice rye bread, toasted
- 1 banana, sliced

Preparation:

Spread almond butter on toast, then Top with banana slices.

CHOCOLATE PEANUT BUTTER OATMEAL

This chocolate peanut butter-style oatmeal tastes just like it heck, it even incorporates some of it into the recipe and is just the ticket to send your taste buds into ecstasy.

Ingredients:

- 3/4 cup (60 g) old fashioned oats
- 3/4 cup milk or water
- 2 egg whites
- 1 tsp cocoa powder
- Cinnamon to taste
- 1/2 chocolate peanut
- 1 tsp (5 g) mini chocolate chips
- 1 tsp (5 g) Reese's peanut butter chips
- 1 tbsp natural peanut butter

Preparation :

Microwave oats and water or milk in a microwave-safe bowl for about 2-1/2 minutes . Add 2 egg whites and whisk until completely mixed in. Microwave for another 45 seconds Add cocoa powder and mix. Add Stevia and cinnamon into small squares. Top with chocolate chips, peanut butter chips, and natural peanut butter.

LOW-CARB PANCAKES

These pancakes fit right into your nutrition program. Make some today!

Ingredients :

- Whole organic egg 1 egg
- Unsweetened almond milk 1/8 cup
- 2 tbsp instant oats

Preparation:

Mix all the ingredients then put into a waffle maker .Cook as you cook a normal pancake and finally top 1-2 tbsp coconut oil and 1 tbsp pure maple.

APPLE & ALMOND MUESLI

An easy recipe to start your day , full of fibers and carbohydrates all you need to stop sleeping catabolism and fill up your muscles.

Ingredients:

- 1/2 cup old-fashioned rolled oats
- 1/2 cup 1% low-fat milk
- 1 apple, cored and chopped

- 2 tablespoons sliced almonds
- 2 teaspoons honey

Preparation :

Combine oats and milk in a small bowl. Let stand 7 minutes. Stir in apple, almonds, and honey.

MORNING BREAKFAST SHAKE

Need a powerful morning punch? Peanut butter? Good. Berries? Good. Oatmeal? Really good! Really, what's not to love about this shake? With a healthy dose of healthy fats, vitamin C, fiber, and protein, it's a well-rounded meal in a glass.

Ingredients:

- 1/2 cup old-fashioned rolled oats
- 1/2 cup 1% low-fat milk
- 1 apple, cored and chopped
- 2 tablespoons sliced almonds

- 2 teaspoons honey

Preparation :

Blend all the ingredients and enjoy!

Lunch Recipes

GRILLED CHICKEN CUTLETS WITH SUMMER SUCCOTASH

You'll learn how to put together a chicken recipe that burns fat and calories, helping you to slim down faster. Plus, it only takes 5 minutes to make!

Ingredients :

- 4 thin chicken cutlets
- 1/4 teaspoon each salt and pepper
- 1 tablespoon olive oil
- 1 cup frozen baby lima beans
- 1/2 cup corn
- 1 pint grape tomatoes
- 1 tablespoon grated Parmesan
- 1/2 cup fresh basil leaves

- lemon wedges
- 100-calorie whole-wheat roll

Preparation:

Place a grill pan over high heat. Season the chicken cutlets with each salt and pepper. Grill until cooked through (about 3-4 minutes), turning once. Meanwhile, heat olive oil in a large skillet over medium-high.
Add in baby lima beans, thawed; corn; and tomatoes. Cook, tossing occasionally, until tomatoes burst (about 3-4 minutes). Stir in grated Parmesan and fresh basil leaves, torn. Pair each portion with lemon wedges and a100-calorie whole-wheat roll.

SHAKE WITH HUMMUS SANDWICH

If you are busy! 5 minute recipe which is very easy to prepare and low in calories.

Ingredients:

- Raspberries
- Kale
- fat-free yogurt

- banana
- honey
- almond butter
- wheat germ
- ice
- whole-grain English muffin,
- hummus

Preparation:

Pair each shake with an open-faced sandwich: 1 tablespoon hummus on 1 toasted whole-grain English muffin.

WHITE BEAN & HERB HUMMUS WITH CRUDITES

It only takes five minutes to whip up a batch of this flavorful, fiber-rich version in your own kitchen.

Ingredients:

- 1/4 cup canned white beans, rinsed and drained
- 1 tablespoon chopped chives
- 1 tablespoon lemon juice

- 2 teaspoons olive oil
- Assorted raw vegetables, such as chopped broccoli florets, sliced green and red peppers, and baby carrots

Preparation:

Combine beans, chives, lemon juice, and oil in a small bowl, mash with a fork until smooth. Serve with 1/2 cup raw vegetables, such as cucumbers, carrots, sugar snap peas, bell peppers, broccoli, and grape tomatoes.

BBQ TURKEY BURGERS

This fresh spin on burgers is a delicious new way to cut back on beef and eat more turkey, an excellent source of lean protein and a good weight-loss food.

Ingredient:

- 1 pound ground dark-meat turkey
- 1 garlic clove, minced
- 1/2 teaspoon paprika
- 1/4 teaspoon ground cumin
- Pinch of kosher salt
- 1/4 teaspoon freshly ground black pepper

- 4 slices sweet onion, grilled
- 1/4 cup barbecue sauce
- 4 (1.6-oz) sesame seed buns, toasted

Preparation :

In medium bowl, gently mix together turkey, garlic, paprika, and cumin, form turkey into 4 (4-inch) patties; season with salt and pepper. Heat grill to medium-high; cook, turning once, until burgers are just cooked through (about 7 minutes per side). Serve with desired toppings and buns.

CURRIED EGG SALAD SANDWICH

This egg salad recipe, a zesty twist on a classic, offers a healthy new way to work eggs into lunchtime. The low-fat Greek yogurt used in place of mayo dials down the fat and calories, while the curry powder provides a jolt of antioxidants.

Ingredients:

- 2 hard-cooked eggs, chopped
- 2 tablespoons plain Greek-style low-fat yogurt

- 2 tablespoons chopped red bell pepper
- 1/4 teaspoon curry powder
- 1/8 teaspoon salt
- 1/8 teaspoon pepper
- 2 slices rye bread, toasted
- 1/2 cup fresh spinach
- 1 orange

Preparation :

Combine eggs, yogurt, bell pepper, curry powder, salt, and pepper, in a small bowl; stir well.

Place spinach on rye bread, top with egg salad, and serve the orange on the side.

HAM SLICED PEAR & SWISS SANDWICH

This recipe is drooling with flavors and textures: Swiss cheese, pear, lean ham, yogurt-dill sauce, and pumpernickel bread. And it's loaded with filling fiber! One sandwich provides nearly one-third of your recommended daily intake of fiber, with the pear alone providing 15%.

Ingredients:

- 1 tablespoon plain Greek-style low-fat yogurt
- 1/4 teaspoon dried dill
- 2 slices pumpernickel bread
- 1 ounce lean sliced ham
- 1 small pear, thinly sliced
- 1 ounce slice Swiss cheese

Preparation :

Combine yogurt and dill in a small bowl, stirring until blended. Spread yogurt mixture on bread slices. Top 1 bread slice with ham, half of pear slices, cheese, and remaining bread slice. Serve with remaining pear slices on the side.

MIDDLE EASTERN RICE SALAD

This 20-minute recipe, which works equally well as a side or a stand-alone meal, is filled to the brim with nutritious ingredients. When it comes to fat burning, though, they're all outshined by the chickpeas.

Ingredient:

- 2 tablespoons olive oil
- 1/2 Vidalia or other sweet onion, thinly sliced (about 3/4 cup)
- 1 (16-ounce) can chickpeas, rinsed and drained
- 1/2 teaspoon ground cumin
- 1/4 teaspoon salt
- Freshly ground black pepper
- 3 cups cooked brown rice
- 1/2 cup chopped pitted dates
- 1/4 cup chopped fresh mint
- 1/4 cup chopped fresh parsley

Preparation:

Heat oil in a large nonstick skillet over medium-high heat. Add onion, and cook, stirring often, about 5 minutes or until onion begins to brown. Remove from heat, and stir in chickpeas, cumin, and salt then season to taste with freshly ground black pepper. Combine rice, onion-chickpea mixture, dates, mint, and parsley in a large bowl and toss well until thoroughly combined. Serve warm or at room temperature.

ENERGY-REVVING QUINOA

Quinoa is one of the trendiest foods around, and for good reason: This earthy whole grain, which hails from South America, is packed with protein and fiber a perfect combination for those who are looking to stay energized and keep their metabolism humming.

Ingredient:

- 1 cup cooked quinoa
- 1/3 cup canned low-sodium black beans, drained and rinsed
- 1 small tomato, chopped
- 1 scallion, sliced
- 1 teaspoon olive oil
- 1 teaspoon fresh lemon juice
- Pinch of salt
- Pinch of freshly ground black pepper

Preparation:

In a medium bowl, gently toss all ingredients to combine.

PAN-GRILLED SALMON WITH PINEAPPLE SALSA

Lean protein is essential to any successful weight-loss plan. And there's no better source of lean protein than salmon, which has the added benefit of being filled with monounsaturated fats.

Ingredients:

- 1 cup chopped fresh pineapple
- 2 tablespoons finely chopped red onion
- 2 tablespoons chopped cilantro
- 1 tablespoon rice vinegar
- 1/8 teaspoon ground red pepper
- Cooking spray
- 4 (6-ounce) salmon fillets (about 1/2-inch thick)
- 1/2 teaspoon salt

Preparation:

Combine first 5 ingredients (through pepper) in a bowl; set aside.

Heat a nonstick grill pan coated with cooking spray over medium-high heat. Sprinkle fish with salt. Cook fish 4 minutes on each side or until it flakes easily when tested with a fork. Top with salsa.

Dinner Recipes

GREEK YOGURT AND CEREAL

Greek yogurt is loaded with healthy bacteria known as probiotics, which perform a host of positive functions for your intestinal health and aid in digestion.

Ingredients:

- 2 cups Greek yogurt
- 2 cups Cereal of your choice

Preparation :

Mix the ingredients and have a good meal !

MAC AND SAUCE CHEESE:

This is a low calorie recipe with a lot of protein , to end your day with .

Ingredients:

- 1/4 cup grated cheedar cheese
- 1 tbsp coconut flour
- 1 tsp powdered cheddar (optional but adds great flavor)
- Garlic salt to taste
- Italian seasoning to taste
- Dry parsley or basil to taste

Preparation:

Cook four servings of the pasta of your choice.Mix all of the sauce ingredients into a bowl. Bring sauce to a simmer and continue to stir until all of the components are well combined. Add the sauce to your pasta, season as desired, and presto! You're done.

BAKED POTATO OATMEAL

Oatmeal with turkey bacon, cheddar cheese, and red potatoes, this dish is a savoury mountain of a meal

Ingredient:

- cooked rolled oats: 1/4 cup
- cubed red potatoes: 100 g (approx. 1/3 cup)
- natural turkey bacon: 2 slices (uncured, nitrate-free, from leg meat)
- reduced-fat shredded cheddar cheese: 1 tbsp
- 2% greek yogurt: 2 tbsp
- chopped green onion: to garnish
- garlic, sea salt, and pepper: to taste

Preparation:

Cook rolled oats as directed.Set oven to 410 degrees F.

Chop red potatoes into pieces and season with garlic, sea salt, and pepper then bake in the oven for about 20 minutes or until soft.Cook turkey bacon in a nonstick skillet while the potatoes are baking in the oven. Once the bacon has finished cooking, allow it to slightly cool and harden. Then, chop the bacon into pieces to create "bacon bits." and add the chopped red potatoes, bacon bits, Greek yogurt and shredded cheddar cheese to the cooked oatmeal.Garnish with freshly chopped green onion and finally season to taste with sea salt and pepper.

CHICKEN AND BROCCOLI

Ditch the cream of chicken soup, butter, and mayonnaise, and try this heart-healthy take on a family classic! It's good for your muscles and easy on your taste buds.

Ingredients:

- 15 oz cooked chicken breast
- 1-1/2 cup 2% Greek yogurt
- 1 cup chicken broth (Add more if you find it too dry, but be careful not to make it "soupy")
- 1 cup reduced-fat mozzarella
- 2 cups cooked quinoa & brown rice mix
- 2 cups raw broccoli, chopped
- 1/4 cup red onion
- 1/2 cup crushed amaranth flakes, wheat breadcrumbs, or panko crumbs
- 1 tbsp Italian seasoning
- Sea salt & pepper to taste

Preparation :

Set oven to 375 degrees Fahrenheit. Cook chicken breasts in a non-stick skillet with no seasoning, or boil the chicken breasts in water then tear the chicken into pieces and set aside. In a bowl, mix chicken, broccoli, brown rice, red onions, Greek yogurt, chicken broth, mozzarella, and Italian seasoning. Evenly divide among the jars or place it all in a large casserole dish, top with wheat breadcrumbs or amaranth flakes and bake for 25 minutes.

GREEK LENTIL SOUP WITH TOASTED PITA

The dish is full of satiating lentils, which provide more than one-third of the recommended daily intake of protein and more than half the recommended intake of protein

Ingredients:

- 1 tablespoon olive oil
- 2 celery stalks, chopped
- 2 carrots, peeled and chopped
- 1 onion
- 2 garlic cloves, minced
- 2 teaspoons dried oregano
- 1/2 teaspoon salt

- 1/2 teaspoon pepper
- 8 cups water
- 1 cup dry lentils
- 2 tablespoons fresh lemon juice (about 1 lemon)
- 4 whole-grain pitas, each cut into 4 triangles and toasted

Preparation:

Heat oil in a large Dutch oven over medium heat then add celery, carrot, onion, garlic, oregano, salt, and pepper; cook 5 minutes. Add the water and lentils. Simmer, partially covered, 15 minutes With a hand blender or potato masher, puree soup until semi-smooth and thick. Drizzle with lemon juice; serve with toasted pita triangles.

EGG AND RICE SALAD

This 10-minute salad-to-go combines fresh flavors and colors from green beans, a hard-boiled egg, plums, walnuts, and brown rice.

Brown rice is a hearty, fiber-packed grain that's low in calories and high in resistant starch. A protein-packed hard-boiled egg and walnuts, which contain healthy omega-3 fats, pair together to help keep you full.

Ingredients:

- 1/2 cup cooked brown rice
- 1 cup cooked green beans, roughly chopped (3 oz)
- 1 ripe plum, thinly sliced (3 oz)
- 2 tablespoons (1/2 oz) chopped walnuts
- 1 hard-cooked egg, sliced
- 1 teaspoon sesame oil
- 2 tablespoons fresh lime juice
- 1/4 teaspoon kosher salt
- Freshly ground black pepper, to taste

Preparation:

Combine rice, beans, plum, walnuts, and egg in a portable container. Drizzle with sesame oil, lime juice, salt, and pepper; toss gently to combine. Refrigerate up to 2 days.

Snacks And Desserts Recipes

CHOCOLATE-DIPPED BANANA BITES

Dessert doesn't have to erase a healthy meal! The bananas in this easier-than-pie dessert—all you need is a knife and a microwave—are a rich source of resistant starch, a type of healthy carbohydrate that helps you burn calories and eat less.

Ingredients:

- 2 tablespoons semisweet chocolate chips
- 1 small banana, peeled and cut into 1-inch chunks

Preparation:

Place chocolate chips in a heavy-duty zip-top plastic bag or small microwave-safe bowl. Microwave at HIGH 1 minute or until chocolate melts. Dip banana pieces in chocolate.

HONEY GRAPEFRUIT WITH BANANA

Trying to trim down or stay slim? You can't go wrong with this tangy tropical fruit salad, perfect for breakfast or as a colourful side dish at brunch. Grapefruit is one of the best foods for weight loss, studies show—perhaps because of the effect it has on insulin, a fat-storage hormone.

Ingredients:

- 1 (24-ounce) jar refrigerated red grapefruit sections (about 2 cups)
- 1 cup sliced banana (about 1)
- 1 tablespoon fresh chopped mint
- 1 tablespoon honey

Preparation :

Drain grapefruit sections, reserving 1/4 cup juice.Combine grapefruit sections, juice, and remaining ingredients in a medium bowl and toss gently to coat. Serve immediately, or cover and chill.

MINI ICE-CREAM CAKES

These fun little cakes are the perfect shade of pink for a little girl's birthday—or just for fun. Use any ice cream or frozen yogurt flavor to tailor it to the guest of honor's preference. You can assemble and freeze the cakes up to a day in advance.

Ingredients:

- Cooking spray
- 1 cup sugar
- 1/3 cup butter, softened
- 2 large eggs
- 1 2/3 cups all-purpose flour
- 1 teaspoon baking powder
- 1/4 teaspoon baking soda
- 1/4 teaspoon salt
- 1 cup low-fat buttermilk
- 1 teaspoon vanilla extract
- 1/4 teaspoon almond extract
- 3 cups low-fat strawberry ice cream, softened
- 1 1/2 cups fat-free frozen whipped topping, thawed
- 1 tablespoon red maraschino cherry juice (optional)
- 12 red maraschino cherries with stems, drained

Preparation:

Preheat oven to 350°.

Coat a 15 x 10-inch jelly-roll pan with cooking spray; line bottom of pan with wax paper. Coat wax paper with cooking spray; set aside.

Place sugar and butter in a large bowl; beat with a mixer at medium speed 5 minutes or until well blended. Add eggs, 1 at a time, beating well after each addition.

Lightly spoon flour into dry measuring cups; level with a knife. Combine flour, baking powder, baking soda, and salt, stirring well with a whisk. Add flour mixture and buttermilk alternately to sugar mixture, beginning and ending with flour mixture; mix after each addition. Beat in extracts. Pour batter into prepared pan. Sharply tap pan once on counter to remove air bubbles. Bake at 350° for 20 minutes or until a wooden pick inserted in center comes out clean. Cool in pan 10 minutes on a wire rack; remove from pan. Carefully peel off wax paper; cool completely on wire rack. Place cake on a large platter or cutting board; refrigerate until cold (about 2 hours).

Spread ice cream evenly over top of cake; cover with plastic wrap. Freeze until firm (6 hours to overnight).

Uncover cake. Cut cake with a 2-inch round cutter into 24 cake rounds. Discard scraps. Working quickly, place one cake round, ice cream side up, in a paper muffin cup liner; top with another cake round, ice cream side down. Repeat procedure with remaining cake rounds to form 12 filled ice-cream cakes.

Combine whipped topping and cherry juice, if desired. Top each cake with 2 tablespoons whipped topping; arrange 1 maraschino cherry on each cake. Freeze until ready to serve. Let ice-cream cakes stand at room temperature 5 minutes before serving.

PEANUT BUTTER-AND-JELLY SANDWICH COOKIE

Peanut butter cookies make the perfect base for a layer of sweet strawberry spread. Serve these sweet-and-salty cookies for an afternoon snack or a sweet lunchbox surprise.

Ingredients:

- 1/4 cup margarine, softened
- 1/4 cup no-sugar-added creamy peanut butter

- 1/2 cup "measures-like-sugar" calorie-free sweetener
- 1/4 cup sugar
- 2 large egg whites
- 1 teaspoon vanilla extract
- 1 3/4 cups all-purpose flour
- 1 teaspoon baking soda
- 1/8 teaspoon salt
- Cooking spray
- 3/4 cup low-sugar strawberry spread

Preparation:

Preheat oven to 350°.

Beat margarine and peanut butter with a mixer at medium speed until creamy. Gradually add sweetener and sugar, beating well. Add egg whites and vanilla; beat well. Combine flour, soda, and salt in a small bowl, stirring well. Gradually add flour mixture to creamed mixture, beating well.

Shape dough into 40 (1-inch) balls. Place balls 2 inches apart on baking sheets coated with cooking spray. Flatten cookies into 2-inch circles using a flat-bottomed glass. Bake at 350° for 8 minutes or until lightly browned. Cool slightly on pans; remove, and let cool completely on wire racks.

Spread about 1 1/2 teaspoons strawberry spread on the bottom of each of 20 cookies; top with remaining cookies.

CHOCOLATE BANANA

For those times when you're craving the classic combination of sweet cocoa and fruit, reach for this recipe. It's a tasty, pre-bedtime snack that you'll enjoy .

Ingredients:

- ½ Cup on fat greek yogurt
- 1 Medium banana
- 1 Dash grated dark chocolate

Preparation:

Slice one medium banana then using a small spoon, apply the chocolate cream onto each slice. Sprinkle with a dash of grated dark chocolate.

VANILLA COOKIES

Bring the holiday cheer without packing on the pounds!

Ingredients:

- 1/3 cup butter
- 1/4 cup brown sugar
- 2 whole eggs
- 1/2 tsp vanilla extract
- 1/2 cup flour
- 1/4 tsp salt
- 1/2 tsp cinnamon
- 1/2 tsp nutmeg
- 6 scoops Grenade Hydra 6 Killa Vanilla
- 1/2 tsp baking soda
- 3/4 cup oats

Preparation :

In a medium bowl, combine butter and brown sugar; Beat in eggs one at a time, then stir in vanilla. In a separate bowl, combine flour, protein powder, baking soda, salt, nutmeg, and cinnamon. Stir into the first mixture then mix in oats. Cover and chill dough for at least one hour. Preheat the oven to 375 F. Grease a cookie sheet with coconut oil, and roll dough balls to place on the sheet. Flatten each cookie with a large fork; Bake 8-10 minutes in preheated oven. Allow cookies to cool on baking sheet for 5 minutes before transferring them onto a wire rack to cool completely.

CREAMY SWEET POTATO DIP

This sweet and spicy snack will rev your metabolism with chipotle chili powder, while the sweet potato fills you up with RS. Speed prep time by using the sweet potato you batch-cooked earlier in the week.

Ingredients:

- 1/2 whole wheat pita, split and cut into 8 pieces
- 1/3 cup roasted mashed sweet potato
- 1 tablespoons plain Greek-style low-fat yogurt
- 1/4 teaspoon honey
- 1/8 teaspoon dried chipotle chile powder
- 1/8 teaspoon salt

Preparation :

Preheat oven to 350°. Arrange pita pieces on a baking sheet; bake at 350° for 10 minutes until crisp. While pita bakes, combine sweet potato, yogurt, honey, chile powder, and salt in a small bowl; stir with a fork until smooth. Serve with warm pita chips.

PEANUT BUTTER BALLS

This recipe provides a healthy source of carbs, protein, and fat. These are easily transportable balls as well, making it ideal for those who are looking for something to snack on at work or during class.

Ingredients:

- 2 cups peanut butter
- 1 scoop chocolate or vanilla protein powder
- 3/4 cup raw oatmeal
- 1 cup crisp rice cereal
- 1/4 cup honey

Preparation:

Microwave the peanut butter on low for about 30 seconds until slightly melted (not runny though).Stir in the honey and protein powder ;once mixed, add in raw oats and crisp rice cereal. Form into balls and then place in the fridge to harden overnight. Note that if you prefer harder/softer peanut butter balls, you can adjust the volumes of the ingredients until your desired texture is reached.

HOME MADE GRANOLA BARS

These are easy and simple to prepare granola bars, full of complex carbs that will nourish your body without making you fat.

Ingredients:

- 2 cups Dry Oatmeal
- 1 cup Honey
- 1 cup Natural Peanut Butter
- 1/4 cup Whole Flax Seed
- 1/4 cup Chopped Almonds
- 1/8 cup Dried Blueberries (Optional)

Preparation:

Melt together honey and peanut butter on low heat. Add in Oatmeal and mix well then mix in other ingredients, stirring to prevent burning. Put mixture in a baking pan and place in freezer until firm cut into small squares.

www.ingramcontent.com/pod-product-compliance
Lightning Source LLC
Chambersburg PA
CBHW071131280526
45787CB00003B/1241